Ameni Jerbi

Atypical aspects of antinuclear antibodies

Ameni Jerbi

Atypical aspects of antinuclear antibodies

Study of atypical aspects of antinuclear antibodies by indirect immunofluorescence on Hep2 cells

ScienciaScripts

Cover image: www.ingimage.com

This book is a translation from the original published under ISBN 978-620-6-71992-2.

Publisher:
Sciencia Scripts
is a trademark of
Dodo Books Indian Ocean Ltd. and OmniScriptum S.R.L publishing group

120 High Road, East Finchley, London, N2 9ED, United Kingdom
Str. Armeneasca 28/1, office 1, Chisinau MD-2012, Republic of Moldova, Europe
Printed at: see last page
ISBN: 978-620-8-05613-1

Table of contents

INTRODUCTION

Antinuclear antibodies are a heterogeneous group of autoantibodies (auto-Abs) directed against a wide variety of antigens of the normal constituents of the cell nucleus, and sometimes of the cytoplasm (nucleic acids, proteins or complexes of both). The interest in AANs lies in the diagnostic value of some of them for the diagnosis of connectivites and certain organ-specific or non-organ-specific autoimmune diseases.

The search for these autoantibodies is carried out in two stages: a 1ère screening stage using an indirect immunofluorescence technique (IFI) on Hep-2 cells, and if the screening is positive, it is followed by a 2ème identification stage of antigenic targets using other immunological techniques (Immunodot, ELISA, RIA, Immunodiffusion...). The use of Hep-2 cells as a substrate for NAA research has heightened awareness that cytoplasmic and mitotic cellular fluorescence can also be recognized, with or without nuclear fluorescence (1). According to the 1er international consensus on standardization of AAN nomenclature "International consensus on anti nuclear antibodies staining Patterns" (ICAP), held in Sao Paolo (Brazil) in 2014, it is recommended to combine cytoplasmic fluorescence and that of the mitotic apparatus with nuclear fluorescence when reporting AAN results (2). Several authors therefore propose the name "anti-cell antibodies" instead of AAN, which appears to be restrictive (3) (4).

However, in current practice, the reporting of NAA results lacks standardization between laboratories: a result is often reported as "positive" or "negative" on the basis of nuclear fluorescence alone.

The objectives of this work were to:

-Describe the nuclear, cytoplasmic and mitotic fluorescence aspects observed during the search for ANNs.

-Study the clinical significance of cytoplasmic labelling aspects isolated from or associated with NAAs.

MATERIALS AND METHODS

1. PATIENTS

This is a cross-sectional study in which we counted all requests for NAA research received in our immunology laboratory at CHU Habib Bourguiba in Sfax, over a period of 11 months (January 2021-November 2021).

2. METHODS

2.1. NAA detection by IFI technique on Hep-2 cells

AAN screening was carried out by IFI on Hep-2 cells using the Hep-2 EUROIMMUN® kit (Germany), which enables IgG isotype detection.
The screening dilution adopted was 1/160 in adults and 1/80 in children (<16 years).

If NAA positivity is detected, the serum is titrated from the starting dilution, using a cascade of increasing dilutions. The NAA titre corresponds to the last serum dilution still showing positive fluorescence.

At least 2 readers use a fluorescence microscope to determine the titer and appearance of nuclear, cytoplasmic or mitotic spindle fluorescence.

2.2. Identification of NAA antigenic targets

2.2.1. Testing for native DNA antibodies

Anti-native DNA was detected by ELISA using the EUROIMMUN® Anti-ds-DNA-NcX ELISA kit (Germany), in accordance with the supplier's recommendations. This kit detects IgG anti-native DNA antibodies. Results are expressed in IU/ml (international unit) using a calibration curve constructed from the various calibrators or standards.

A result is considered positive above 100IU/ml.

2.2.2. Testing for antibodies to soluble nuclear antigens

The detection of soluble nuclear antigen Ac was performed by

Immundot technique using the EUROLINE ANA Profile 3 plus DFS kit (EUROIMMUN®, Germany) which allows the detection of Ac of isotype IgG directed against 16 different autoantigens: RNP/Sm, Sm, SSA (native), Ro-52, SSB, Scl-70, PM-Scl, Jo-1, B centromere, PCNA, dsDNA (double-stranded), nucleosomes, histones, ribosomal protein P, AMA-M2 and DFS70.

The strips are read by a scanner (EUROLineScan) and the result is semi-quantitative (+: weakly positive; ++: positive; +++: strongly positive).

3. STATISTICAL ANALYSIS

Statistical analysis was performed using SPSS.22.0 software.

RESULTS

A total of 2952 NAA search requests were received during the study period.

NAA testing revealed 2,572 positive results (87%) and 380 negative results (13%); an average of 233 positive results per month.

1. EPIDEMIOLOGICAL CHARACTERISTICS OF PATIENTS WITH ANTI-NUCLEAR ANTIBODIES POSITIVE

1.1. Patient distribution by age

The age of AAN-positive patients ranged from 1 to 94 years, with an average age of 38. The age groups most concerned were those aged between 40 and 60, followed by those aged between 20 and 40 **(figure 1)**.

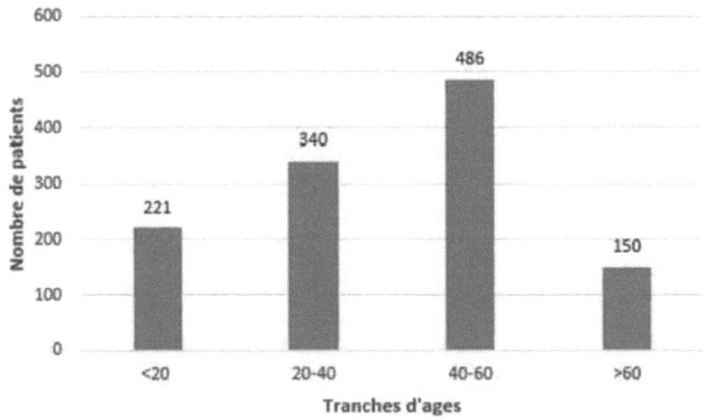

Figure 1: Distribution of AAN-positive patients by age group

1.2. Patient distribution by gender

In our series, there was a clear predominance of females: 1936 females (75%) and 636 males (25%), i.e. a sex ratio (f/h) of 3/1 **(figure 2).**

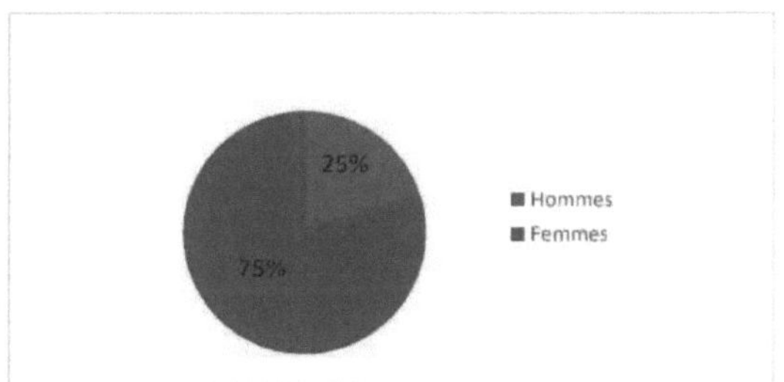

Figure 2: Distribution of NAA-positive patients by sex

NAA-positive women were younger (mean age 37.6 years) than men (mean age 41.4 years), with no statistically significant difference (p=0.128).

1.3. Patient distribution by clinical department

The majority of our patients came from the departments of internal medicine (21%), pediatrics (8.7%), rheumatology (7.5%), neurology (7%), clinical hematology (6.9%), nephrology (6.7%), dermatology (5.8%) and gastroenterology (2.9%) **(Figure 3)**.

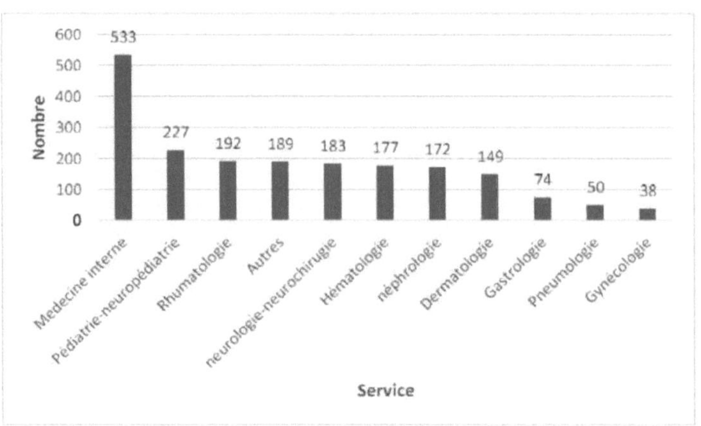

Figure 3: **Distribution of AAN-positive patients by department**

2. IMMUNOLOGICAL STUDY OF POSITIVE ANTINUCLEAR ANTIBODIES

The various aspects of the positive NAAs observed in our series are shown in Figure 4.

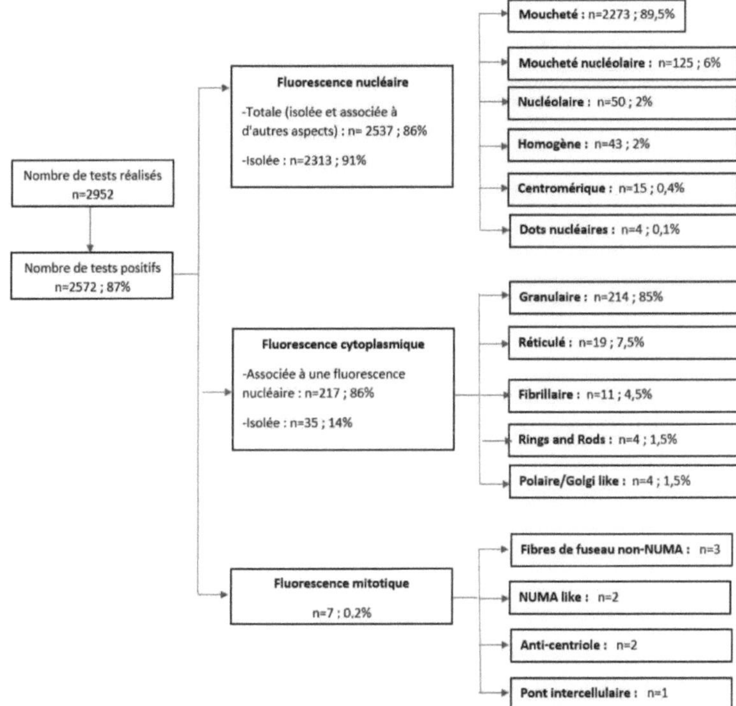

Figure 4: Distribution of the different fluorescence aspects of NAAs in our study

2.1. Nuclear marking aspects

The nuclear fluorescence aspects most frequently observed in our study were: **(figures 5 and 6)**

- Speckled in 89.5% of cases (n=2273)

* Nucleolar speckle in 6% of cases (n=152)

- Nuclear in 2% of cases (n=50)
- Homogenous in 2% of cases (n=43)
- Other aspects were rare in our series, such as the anti centromere (15 cases, 0.4%) and nuclear dots (4 cases, 0.1%).

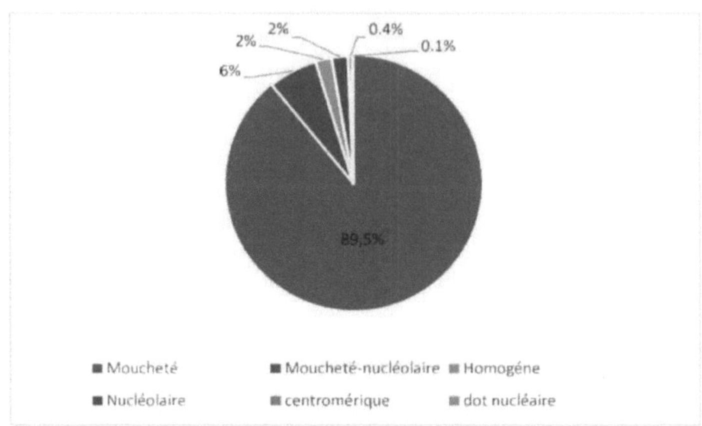

***Figure 5*: Different aspects of nuclear labelling of Hep-2 cells observed in our series**

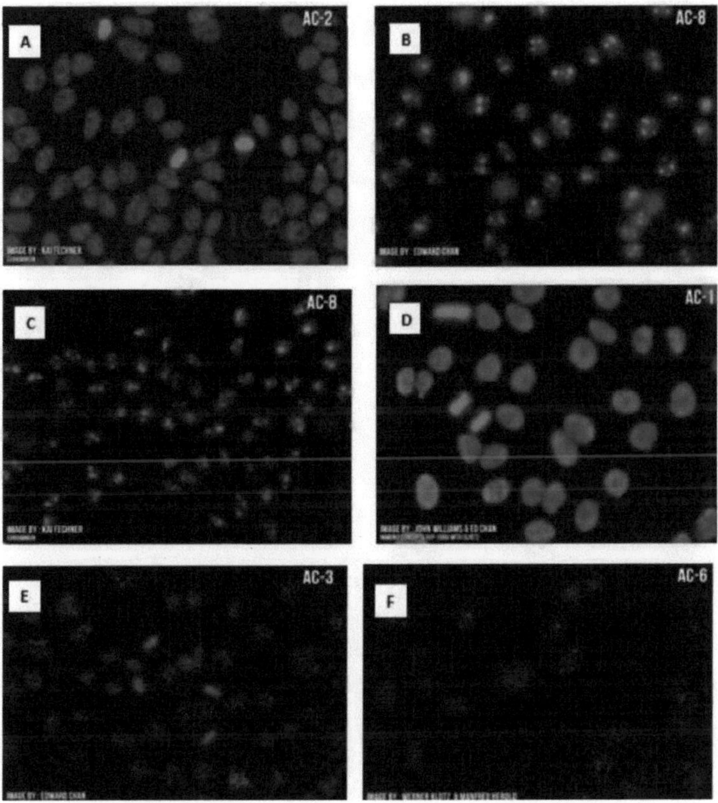

Figure 6: The different aspects of antinuclear antibodies observed in our series by indirect immunofluorescence technique on Hep2 cells:

(A) Speckled appearance: presence of very small, fine grains throughout the nucleoplasm; (B) nucleolar speckled appearance; (C) nucleolar appearance: diffuse fluorescence throughout the nucleolus; (D) homogeneous appearance: even, homogeneous fluorescence throughout the nucleoplasm. Cells in mitosis (metaphase, anaphase and telophase) have their chromatin intensely marked in a homogeneous and hyaline manner; (E) A spect anti centromere: In cells in interphase, presence of around 40 dispersed large grains per cell. In cells in mitosis, these grains are aligned and superimposed on the chromatin; (F) appearance of nuclear dots: Discrete nuclear dots that can be counted (i.e. 6 to 20 nuclear dots per cell corresponding to multiple nuclear dots, i.e. 1 to 6 nuclear dots).

- The most frequently observed titers were: 1/320 (n=844

33%),1/640 (n=591; 23%) and 1/1280 (n=588; 23%).

Titles of 1/160 and 1/80 were less frequent **(figure 7).**

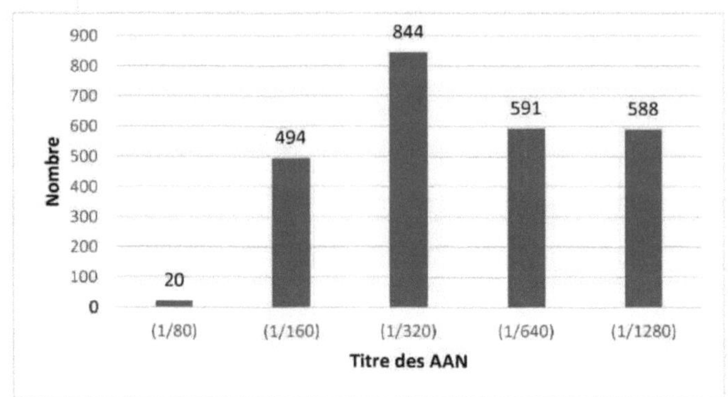

Figure 7: **Distribution of positive anti-nuclear antibody results by titer**

2.2. Aspects of cytoplasmic marking

Cytoplasmic fluorescence of Hep-2 cells was observed in 252 patients, or 8.6% of all sera tested during the study period. This cytoplasmic fluorescence was associated with nuclear labeling in 217 cases (86%) and isolated in 35 cases (14%) **(figure 8).**

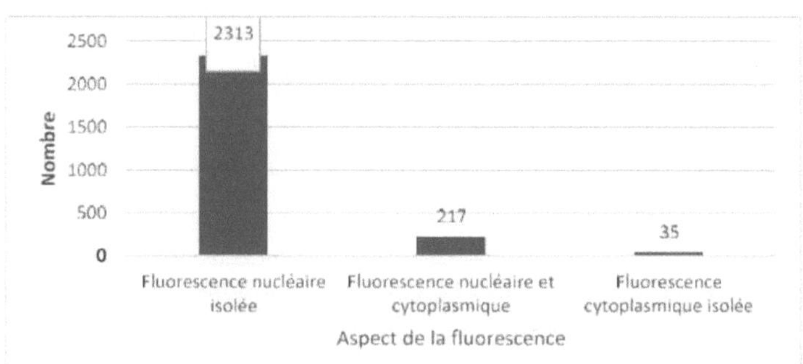

Figure 8: **Association of nuclear and cytoplasmic fluorescence aspects in our series**

The most frequently observed cytoplasmic marking patterns were: granular (214 cases, 85%), reticulated (19 cases, 7.5%), fibrillar (11 cases, 4.5%), rods and rings (4 cases ,1.5%) and polar/golgi-like (4 cases, 1.5%) (figure 9).

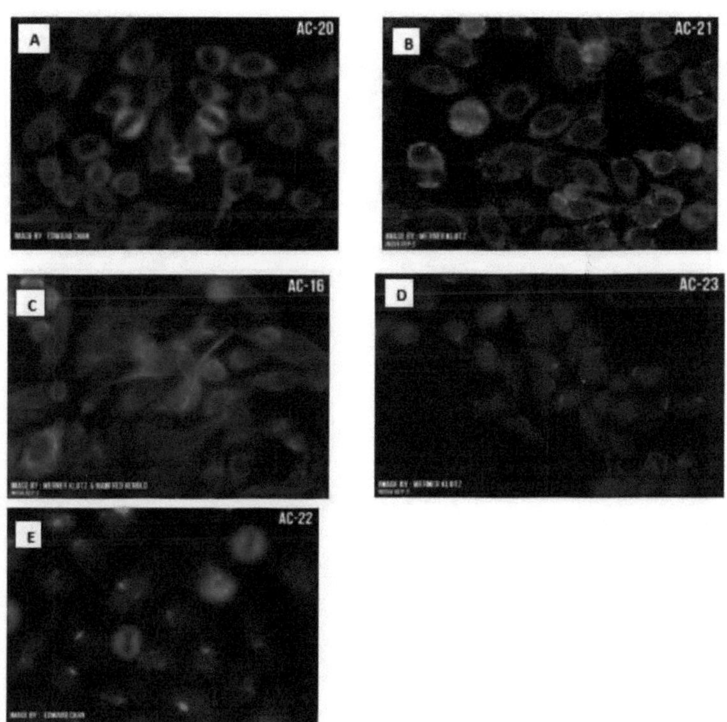

Figure 9: The different aspects of cytoplasmic fluorescence observed in our series:

(A) granular: fine granulations scattered throughout the cytoplasm; (B) reticulated: coarse filamentous and granular marking present throughout the frayed cytoplasm; (C) fibrillar: marking of microtubules and intermediate filaments extending from the periphery of the nucleus; (D) rods and rings: distinct rod and ring structures in the cytoplasm of interphase cells; (E) polar/golgi-like: speckled or granular peri-nuclear (ribbon-like) labeling with polar localization in the cytoplasm.

2.1. Mitotic spindle marking aspects

Mitotic spindle fluorescence was observed in 7 cases (0.2%). The various aspects were: (figure 10)

- Non-NUMA spindle fibers (3 cases)
- NuMA-Iike (2 cases)
- Anti centioles (1 case)
- Intercellular bridge (1 case)

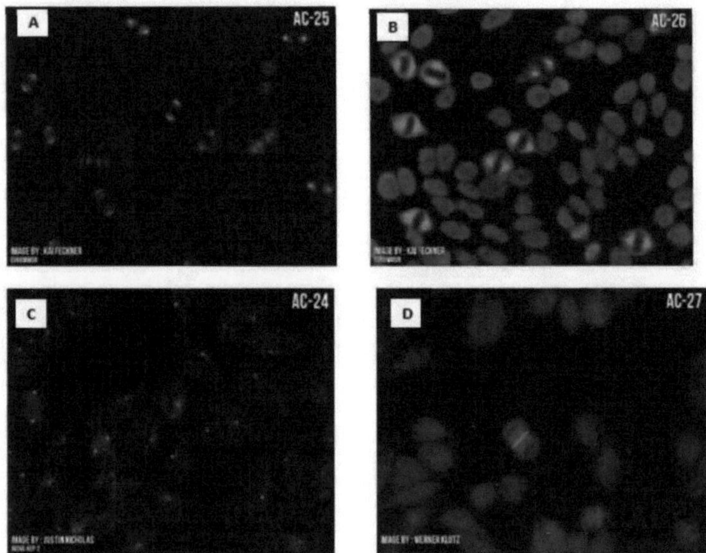

Figure 10: The different aspects of mitotic spindle fluorescence observed in our series: (A) Non NuMA spindle fibers: spindle fiber labeling, (B) Numa-like: speckled nuclear fluorescence with spindle fiber labeling; (C) Anti centrioles; (D) Intercellular bridge.

3. ETUDE DES SIGNIFICATIONS CLINIQUES ASSOCIES AUXA SPECTS DE MARQUAGE CYTOPLASMIQUE

Among 252 cases with cytoplasmic staining associated or not with nuclear fluorescence, clinical information was available for 134 patients (53%). Tables I and II summarize the clinical information for these patients.

Table I: Clinical manifestations associated with the presence of cytoplasmic fluorescence with or without nuclear labeling in patients (n=134)

Different aspects of cytoplasmic fluorescence	*Selected diagnoses and/or associated clinical and biological manifestations*
Granular	***Systemic lupus erythematosus (SLE) (n=17) Rheumatoid arthritis (RA) (n=4) Gougerot Sjogren's syndrome (GSS) (n=1) Anti-phospholipid syndrome (SAPL) (n=1) Scleroderma (n=1) Necrotizing myositis (n=1) Anti-synthetase syndrome (n=1) Polymyositis (n=4) Dermatomyositis (n=1) Suspicion of connectivity (n=7) Events ocular (n=7) Neurological manifestations (n=7) Diffuse interstitial lung disease (n=6)Mucocutaneous manifestations: Dry syndrome (n=8) Events cutaneous (n=9) Joint manifestations (n=15) Hematological manifestations (n=9) Cytolysis and cholestasis (n=4)***

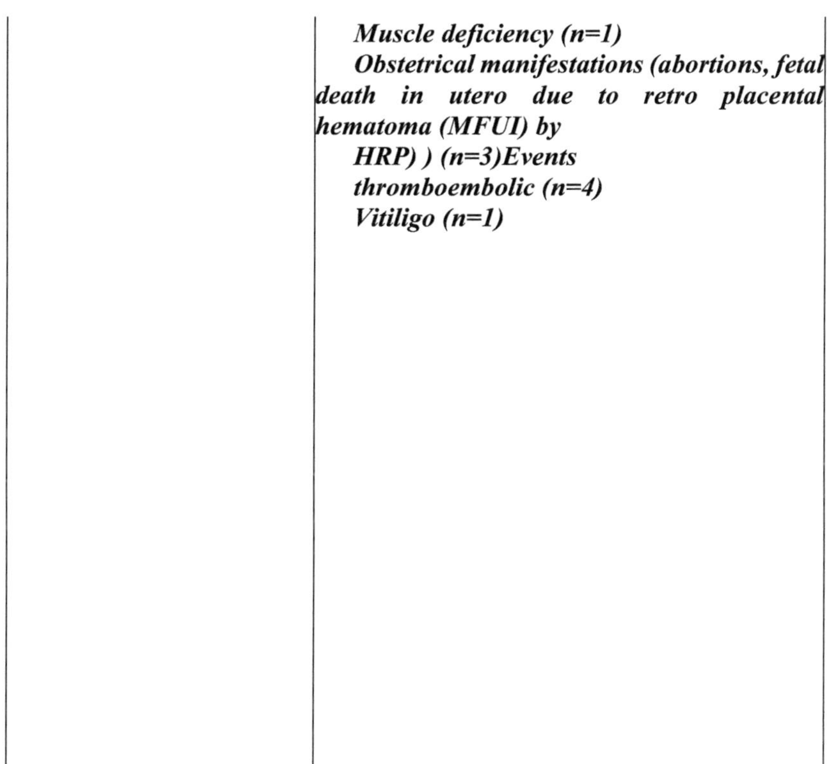

	Muscle deficiency (n=1) *Obstetrical manifestations (abortions, fetal death in utero due to retro placental hematoma (MFUI) by* *HRP)) (n=3)Events* *thromboembolic (n=4)* *Vitiligo (n=1)*

Reticulated	***Primary biliary cirrhosis (CBP) (n=1)CBP+PR (n=1)*** ***LES+S*** ***APL*** ***(n=1)*** ***SGJ*** ***(n=1)*** ***Recurrent miscarriage (n=1)*** ***Dry syndrome (n=2)*** ***Events*** ***joints (n=2)*** ***Thrombocytopenia (n=1)*** ***Raynaud's phenomenon, telangiectasia (n=1)***

Fibrillar	***Myositis (n=1)Stroke (n=1)*** ***Polyarthritis and dry mouth (n=1) Thrombocytopenia, anemia, polyclonal hypogammaglobulinemia (n=3) Autoimmune hypothyroidism (n=1)*** ***Diabetes (n=1)*** ***Recurrent pericarditis (n=1)***

Rings and rods	***Vitiligo (n=1)*** ***Biological inflammatory syndrome (n=1)*** ***Cholestasis (n=1)***

Polar/golgi-like	*Dermatosis annulare (n=1)*

Table II: Clinical manifestations associated with the presence of isolated cytoplasmic fluorescence (n=15)

Isolated cytoplasmic fluorescence patterns	*Selected diagnosis*
Granular	***Dry syndrome (n=3)*** ***Diffuse interstitial lung disease PID (n=2)*** ***LES (n=2)*** ***Necrotizing myositis (n=1)*** ***Anti-synthetase syndrome (n=1)PR (n=1)*** ***Inflammatory disease of the nervous system central (n=1)*** ***Muscle deficiency (n=1)MFIU HRP (n=1)*** ***Thrombocytopenia (n=1)***
Fibrillar	***Diabetes (n=1)***
Reticulated	***CBP + PR (n=1)***

The presence of cytoplasmic fluorescence with or without nuclear labeling was associated with various clinical situations such as:

"Connectivity:

Connectivity was confirmed in 20 patients (19%): 17 cases of lupus, 2 cases of Gougerot Sjogren's syndrome (GSS) and 1 case of scleroderma.

Connectivitis was suspected in 7 patients (6 cases of SLE and 1 single case).

SGS).

- **Rheumatoid arthritis**

Four patients were being followed for rheumatoid arthritis (RA)

- **Inflammatory myopathies**

Four patients had polymyositis, 1 patient had a muscle deficit, and another patient had dermatomyositis.

Interestingly, we noted the presence of a particular cytoplasmic fluorescence without nuclear labelling in 2 patients. This was complemented by a dot myositis test, which was positive for SRP antibodies in one patient and for Jol antibodies in the other. Taken together, the clinical, biochemical and immunological data led to the diagnoses of necrotizing myopathy and anti-synthetase syndrome in the 2 patients respectively.

- **Diffuse interstitial lung disease**

Cytoplasmic labeling was observed in 6 patients followed for diffuse interstitial lung disease (DILD).

- **Hepatopathies**

The diagnosis of primary biliary cirrhosis (PBC) was confirmed in one patient and suspected in 4 others, given the presence of cytolysis and choie stasis.

We had another interesting case of a patient with RA for whom NAA had been requested. The appearance on IFI was that of cross-linked cytoplasmic staining suggestive of anti-mitochondrial DNA. Further investigation confirmed the presence of M2-type anti-mitochondrial antibodies and the diagnosis of PBC associated with RA.

- **Joint manifestations**

AANs were requested in front of demonstrations

polyarthralgia in 18 patients.

- **Neurological manifestations**

Neurological manifestations were present in 7 patients:

4 cases of stroke, 2 cases of myelitis and 1 case of inflammatory disease of the central nervous system.

- **Ocular manifestations**

Ocular manifestations were observed in 7 patients: uveitis (5 cases), ptosis (1 case) and retrobulbar optic neuropathy (1 case).

- **Hematological manifestations**

Eight patients had thrombocytopenia, 3 had anemia, and one had macrophagic activation syndrome.

- **Mucocutaneous manifestations**

Mucocutaneous manifestations were observed in 19 patients, in the form of dry occulo-buccal syndrome (10 cases) or mucocutaneous signs (9 cases).

- **Thrombo-embolic manifestations**

Four patients had deep vein thrombosis (DVT) of different locations (lower limbs (2 cases), central retinal vein (1 case), internal jugular vein (1 case)). Anti-phospholipid syndrome was suspected in one patient.

- **Obstetrical manifestations**

There was one case of fetal death in utero and 2 cases of recurrent miscarriage.

- **Other signs of autoimmunity**

NAAs were requested in 2 cases of vitiligo, one case of autoimmune hypothyroidism and one case of diabetes.

DISCUSSION

AANs are autoantibodies directed against antigenic determinants in the nuclei of the body's cells.

AANs can be observed in the context of non-organ-specific autoimmune diseases (such as SLE, Gougerot Sjogren's syndrome, systemic scleroderma, mixed connectivitis, dermatomyositis...) or in the course of certain organ-specific autoimmune diseases, in particular autoimmune liver diseases.

They can also be observed in a variety of situations, such as cancer, acute or chronic leukemia, infection (with parvovirus B19 or Epstein-Barr virus) or even in apparently healthy subjects, with a prevalence of 5 to 30% (5), particularly in pregnant women, women over 40 and elderly subjects.

In general, NAAs are considered a good screening test for connectivites, given their good sensitivity, although they lack specificity.

1. AAN DETECTION METHODS

1.1. The substrate

LTFI is currently the most widely used method for NAA testing. It is a simple, rapid and effective technique, perfectly suited to serial analysis.

LTFI can be performed on several substrates, such as Hep-2 cell cultures or organ sections (liver, rat). The analytical performance of these substrates is not equivalent. Hep-2 cells are the substrate of choice for NAA testing. They are derived from tumor cell cultures (human laryngeal carcinoma; Hep- 2: human epithelial cell line type 2).

Compared with the organ courses (liver, rat) used previously, Hep-2 cells have the advantage of a large nucleus, abundant nuclear antigens, abundant cytoplasm, and cells at different stages of the cell cycle, enabling the detection of NAAs directed against target antigens present only at certain phases of the cell cycle.

Thus, IFI on$_{ce}$ llules H$_{e}$ p-2 is the "gold standard" for AAN screening (6) (7).

1.2. Positivity threshold

The threshold for NAA positivity has long been a subject of debate. The[5] European League against Rheumatism (EULAR) and the American College of Rheumatology have recently set the threshold value for NAA positivity at 1:80 (8).

In practice, however, this threshold needs to be determined by the laboratory in order to better discriminate between healthy subjects and those with connective tissue disease. Several thresholds can be used: 1:40, 1:80, 1:100 , 1:160 and 1:200 (9) (10). But the most commonly used thresholds are 1:80 and 1:100.

In our laboratory, our positivity threshold is set at 1:160 for adults and 1:80 for children, as low NAA positivity in children often reflects an inflammatory or even autoimmune pathology (11).

The chosen positivity threshold influences the AAN positivity rate. For example, the positivity rate in the healthy population is between 25 and 30% for a threshold of 1/40, 10 to 15% at 1/80 and 5% at 1/160 (7,12).

2. AAN POSITIVITY STUDY

2.1. Prevalence of positive NAAs

The prevalence of positive NAAs varies in the literature, not only according to the different reagents used (inter-reagent variability), but also within laboratories using the same reagent (intra-reagent variability: sample dilution, positivity threshold, magnification of the lens used by readers...). (13).

This prevalence varies from 26.7% (14), to 39.7% (15) at a threshold of 1:80 up to 53% (16).

In our study, the prevalence of positive NAAs was 87%, which appears to be high compared with the literature. This could be explained on the one hand by a good pre-test probability. Indeed, the majority of requests for NAA testing in our laboratory came from hospital wards such as internal medicine and rheumatology, where patients are monitored for autoimmune or inflammatory diseases.

The prevalence of positive NAA also depends on the positivity threshold (17). Although we had higher thresholds, we also had a high prevalence of positive NAAs, suggesting that there are geo-epidemiological differences in the prevalence of NAAs. An increase in the prevalence of NAA positivity in recent years has also been suggested. A recent study conducted by the National Survey of Health and Nutrition of Americans in which sera from 14,211 US residents over the age of 12 collected over three periods (1988-1991, 1999-2004 and 2011-2012) were systematically tested for NAA in a laboratory by IFI on HEp-2 cells, and the results correlated with clinical data. The results indicate that there is a clear and statistically significant trend towards an increase in the number of HIV-positive Americans over the years, particularly in the most recent period (from 11% and 11.5% to 15.5%).

More recently, autoantibodies are frequently detected in patients with COVID-19, perhaps reflecting a pathogenic role for immune dysregulation. According to Simone et al, the prevalence of AANs in this population was 33% (18). Peker et al found that 18% of patients with COVID-19 were positive for NAA (19). These studies further support the involvement of SARS-CoV-2 in triggering autoimmunity. However, the causal link between covid-19 and autoimmunity is difficult to establish.

It has been consistently reported that NAAs are more common in women (20.1%) than in men (11.4%), in subjects over 50 years of age (20.5%) than in young people (13%), and in African Americans (18.1%) than in other ethnic groups (20).

In our series, AAN was also more frequent in women. Generally speaking, autoimmune diseases (AIDs) are seen preferentially in women of all ages, but especially in the young. Several mechanisms may account for the aggravating role of estrogens and the beneficial effect of androgens on AIDs. Estrogens increase prolactin and growth hormone secretion, which in turn may play a role in T and B lymphocyte proliferation (21). Androgens, on the other hand, appear to exert mainly inhibitory effects on the immune response in general and autoimmunity in particular, through mechanisms acting directly on cells of the immune system (increased activity of regulatory T lymphocytes) or on certain target organs.

These observations suggest that androgen deficiency may be associated with the development of immunopathological manifestations (22).

2.2. The main aspects of AAN

The appearance observed on IFI reflects the cellular distribution of autoantigens, which may diffuse freely in the cytosol or, on the contrary, be restricted to a particular structure or organelle. The appearance of fluorescence generally points to antigenic specificities.

According to the ICAP consensus (1), 3 types of fluorescence can be observed in Hep-2 cells by IFI, depending on the localization of antigenic targets in the cell: nuclear, cytoplasmic or mitotic (figure 11).

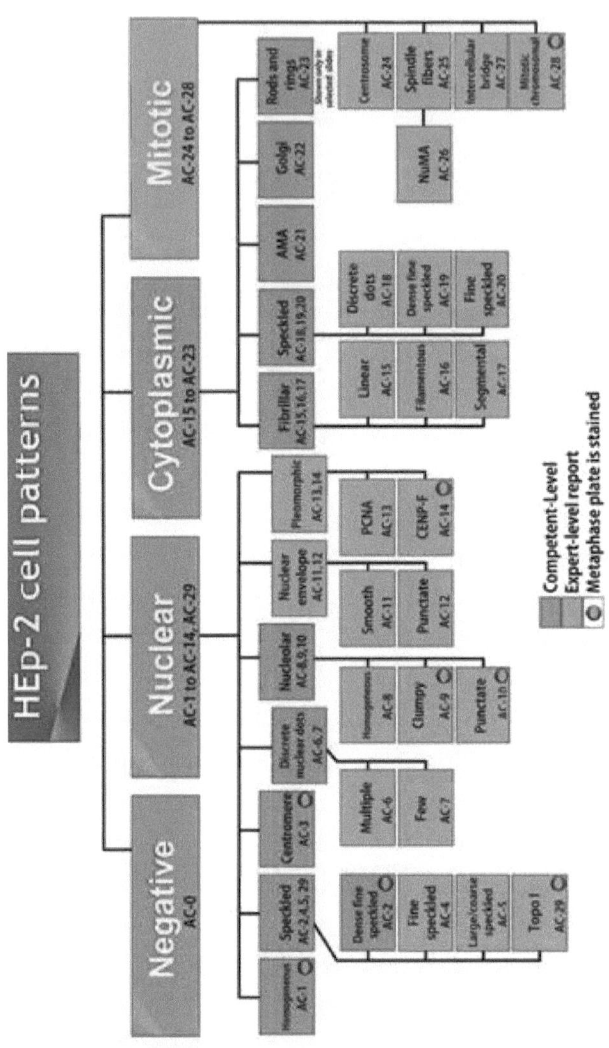

Figure 11: Nomenclature and classification tree of nuclear, cytoplasmic and mitotic fluorescence aspects by indirect immunofluorescence on Hep2 cells.

While some of these mainly nuclear aspects are well described and studied in the literature, others are less well known and often not reported by biologists.

2.2.1. Nuclear fluorescence aspects

Classically, the nuclear fluorescence observed is of the homogeneous, speckled, nucleolar, centromeric type and more rarely in Each of these fluorescence aspects can be observed in isolation or nuclear dots associated with the other aspects.

Homogeneous fluorescence of nuclei can be given by various antigenic specificities such as anti-DNA, anti-nucleosome and anti-histone Ac.

When homogeneous NAA titer is high, there may be peripheral enhancement that must be distinguished from nuclear membrane fluorescence.

- Speckled fluorescence is mainly produced by antibodies to soluble nuclear antigens, also known as anti-ENA ("extractable nuclear antigens") (or anti-ECT for "thymic cell extract"). These antibodies can be directed against a wide variety of antigenic targets identifiable by specific tests (immunodot, ELISA...). In our series, the speckled appearance was the most frequent.
- Homogeneous nucleolar fluorescence is observed in the following major antigenic specificities: PM/Scl, NOR-90, fibrillarin, U3RNP and mainly associated with scleroderma.
- Anti-centromere antibodies can have as antigenic target CENP-A (p17), -B (p80), -C (p140), -D (p50), -F (p400). They are mainly found in the course of the syndrome of

CREST (80 to 100% of cases), but also in Reynolds syndrome (CBP + scleroderma) and various other autoimmune diseases (SLE, Gougerot-Sjogren's, etc.).

2.2.2. Cytoplasmic fluorescence aspects and their clinical significance

The observation of cytoplasmic fluorescence in HEp-2 cell IFI tests for NAA is far from exceptional.

It may be associated with nuclear fluorescence or isolated, and in the latter case may be unrecognized and underestimated.

The prevalence of cytoplasmic fluorescence varies in the literature from 4.9% (23) to 10.3% (24). In our study, cytoplasmic labeling was observed in 8.6% of sera tested. This marking was isolated in 0.8% of cases.

As soon as cytoplasmic fluorescence is considered significant, and not simply background noise, its interpretation will take into account its appearance. The frequency of these different aspects varies from series to series, and we have identified several cytoplasmic aspects in our series:

- Granular cytoplasmic appearance (coarse, fine and diffuse) was more frequent in our patients. It was observed in 63% of patients with cytoplasmic staining, in line with data from an English series which noted its presence with a frequency of 66% (25). This feature has been observed in connective tissue diseases such as SLE and inflammatory myopathies.

- The reticulated aspect was the 2ème aspect observed in terms of frequency in 7% of patients. In our study, it was associated with PBC with M2 anti-mitochondrial antibodies in 2 of 11 patients. Seema Chhabra et al. found this appearance in PBC alone or associated with autoimmune hepatitis (23).

Interestingly, three patients had isolated cytoplasmic fluorescence, which helped to establish the following diagnoses: necrotizing myositis with specific anti-SRP Ac in one case, anti-synthetase syndrome with anti-Jo1 Ac in another, and PBC with M2-type anti-mitochondrial Ac associated with RA in the third patient.

- Fibrillar appearance was rare in our patients. It was not associated with systemic rheumatic autoimmune diseases.

Our data are therefore in line with what has been described in the literature (23).

- An anti-Golgi apparatus appearance with peri-nuclear crescent-shaped cytoplasmic fluorescence was not common in our series (1.5%). This appearance was associated with various pathologies. The significance of these Ac remains unclear and controversial in the literature (26): while some authors associate these Ac with the development of Gougerot syndrome and long-term rheumatic disease (23), others find no pathological association (1). The rare prevalence of this aspect and the heterogeneity of results from one study to another are responsible for these conflicting results.

-The prevalence of Ring and Rods was a low 1.5%. The presence of these Ac was associated with a variety of clinical situations, including vitiligo and cholestasis. In the literature, this appearance is rare (14) and is often reported in

- hepatitis C patients on InterferonZribavirin (14). We had no patients with hepatitis C.

2.2.3. Aspects of mitotic spindle fluorescence

The prevalence of mitotic spindle fluorescence reported in the literature ranges from 0.4% (23) to 1% in the largest cohorts, such as Betancur et al. (16), which included 113,491 requests for AAN.

This aspect is therefore considered one of the rarest in current practice.

(14).

Several aspects can be observed: centrosome, spindle fibers (NuMA-like, and non-NuMA), intercellular bridge, and mitotic chromosome.The NuMA-Iike aspect was the most frequent in our series with a prevalence of 0.06% close to that reported in a Chinese study 0.04% (27). This aspect was more frequent in other studies: 0.7% in a European cohort (28) and 0.4% in the cohort of Betancur et al.(16). The rarity of this aspect and the fact that it is not systematically reported by biologists contribute to the heterogeneity of results.

While many of the fluorescence aspects of the mitotic spindle appear to be of no clinical interest, the NuMA-Iike aspect is attracting the most interest as it has been associated with autoimmune diseases (14).

CONCLUSION

In our study, we recorded all AAN research requests received in our laboratory over a 10-month period. We analyzed the different aspects (nuclear, cytoplasmic and mitotic) observed by IFI in accordance with the I[1] ICAP classification, and studied the clinical significance of cytoplasmic aspects associated or not with nuclear labeling.

The search for NAAs is a frequent motif in clinical biology. The interest in NAAs lies in the diagnostic value of some of them in the diagnosis of connectivites and certain autoimmune diseases, whether or not they are organ-specific. However, in current practice, the reporting of AAN results lacks standardization between laboratories.

In our study, we listed all NAA search requests received by our laboratory over a 10-month period. We analyzed the various aspects of nuclear, cytoplasmic and mitotic fluorescence observed that in accordance with the recommendations of the 1st international consensus on standardization of AAN nomenclature (ICAP 2014). In a 2nd step, we analyzed the clinical meanings of cytoplasmic markings.

Our results showed a high prevalence of AAN, particularly in young women. Unlike mitotic spindle fluorescence, cytoplasmic fluorescence is not uncommon. It was predominantly granular. Reticulated and filamentous aspects were less frequent. Taking account of these particular isolated cytoplasmic aspects, in line with ICAP recommendations, enabled us to supplement with specific explorations and contribute to the clinical diagnosis.

However, our study is limited by sample size, retrospective nature and lack of clinical information.

In conclusion, our results underline the fact that IFI Hep-2 cells is a comprehensive technique that can provide useful data to the clinician. The reporting of NAA results should include nuclear, cytoplasmic and mitotic labeling aspects. In medical practice, the significance of cytoplasmic fluorescence when testing for NAA is not unequivocal. While some aspects have no diagnostic value, others are of real clinical interest and must be recognized and mentioned by the biologist in order to implement NAA identification techniques when necessary, as part of a good clinical-biological collaboration.

REFERENCES

1. Damoiseaux J, von Mühlen CA, Garcia-De La Torre I, Carballo OG, de Melo Cruvinel W, Francescantonio PLC, et al. International consensus on ANA patterns (ICAP): the bumpy road towards a consensus on reporting ANA results. Autoimmun Highlights. 2016;7(1):1.

2. Agmon-Levin N, Damoiseaux J, Kallenberg C, Sack U, Witte T, Herold M, et al. International recommendations for the assessment of autoantibodies to cellular antigens referred to as anti-nuclear antibodies.-Ann Rheum Dis. 2014;73(1):17 23.

3. Damoiseaux J, Andrade LEC, Carballo OG, Conrad K, Francescantonio PLC, Fritzler MJ, et al. Clinical relevance of HEp-2 indirect immuno fluorescent patterns: The International Consensus on ANA patterns (ICAP) perspective. Annals of the Rheumatic Diseases. 2019;78(7):879 89.

4. Chan EKL, Damoiseaux J, Carballo OG, Conrad K, de Melo Cruvinel W, Francescantonio PLC, et al. Report of the First International Consensus on Standardized Nomenclature of Antinuclear Antibody HEp-2 Cell Patterns (ICAP) 2014-2015. Frontiers in Immunology. 2015;6(JUL):1 13.

5. Rita B, Jennifer MA, Danièle A. Impact of antinuclear antibody testing in daily clinical practice. Revue Medicale Suisse. 2021

6. Jetée LM, Peter HS. ANA screening: an old test with new recommendations.Ann Rhcum Dis. 2010;69(8)1420-2

7. Solomon DH, Kavanaugh AJ, Schur PH, Guidelines AC of RAHC on IT. Evidence-based guidelines for the use of immunologic tests:

Antinuclear antibody testing. Arthritis Care & Research. 2002;47(4):434 44.

8. Aringer M, Costenbader K, Daikh D, Brinks R, Mosca M, Ramsey-Goldman R, et al. 2019 European League Against RheumatismZAmerican College of Rheumatology Classification Criteria for Systemic Lupus Erythematosus. Arthritis Rheumatol. 2019;71(9):1400 12.

9. Pashnina IA, Krivolapova IM, Fedotkina TV, Ryabkova VA, Chereshneva MV, Churilov LP, et al. Antinuclear Autoantibodies in Health: Autoimmunity Is Not a Synonym of Autoimmune Disease. Antibodies (Basel). 2021;10(1):9.

10. Naides SJ, Genzen JR, "Abel G, Bashleben C, Ansari MQ. Antinuclear Antibodies Testing Method Variability: A Survey of Participants in the College of American Pathologists of Rheumatology. 2020;47(12):1768 73.

11. Goulvestre C. Antinuclear antibodies. La Presse Médicale. 2006;35(2):287 95.

12. Tozzoli R, Bizzaro N, Tonutti E, Villalta D, Bassetti D, Manoni F, et al. Guidelines for the laboratory use of autoantibody tests in the diagnosis and monitoring of autoimmune rheumatic diseases. Am J Clin Pathol. 2002;117(2):316 24.

13. Albarede S, Guyard A, Daunizeau A, Graeve JD, Pham B-N. Specialized Biochemistry / Immunopathology.2007

14. Nanda R, Gupta P, Patel S, Shah S, Mohapatra E. Uncommon antinuclear antibody patterns as diagnostic indicators. Clin Biochem.

2021;90:28 33.

15. Chauhan R, Jain D, Dorwal P, Roy G, Raina V, Nandi SP. The incidence of immunofluorescence patterns and specific autoantibodies observed in autoimmune patients in a tertiary care center. Eur Ann Allergy Clin Immunol.2019;51(4):165 73.

16. Betancur JF, Londoflo A, Estrada VE, Puerta SL, Osorno SM, Loaiza A, et al. Uncommon patterns of antinuclear antibodies recognizing mitotic spindle apparatus antigens and clinical associations. Medicine (Baltimore). 2018;97(34):e11727.

17. Tomasik T, et al. Analysjs of the impact of sex and age on the variation in the prevalence of antinuclear autoantibodies in Polish population: a nationwide observational, cross-sectional study. Rheumatol Int. 2022;42(2):261 71.

18. Pascolini S, Vannini A, Deleonardi G, Ciordinik M, Sensoli A, Carletti I, et al. COVID-19 and Immunological Dysregulation: Can Autoantibodies be Useful? Clin Transl Sci. 2021;14(2):502 8.

19. Beenet L. Role of antinuclear antibodies in COVID-19 patients. J ImmunolMethods. 2022;502:113215.

20. Gregg ED, Christine GP, Clarice RW, Caroll ACo, Jesse W, Darryl CZ et al. Increasing Prevalence of Antinuclear Antibodies in the United States Arthrite Rheumatol. 2020

21. Huck S, Zouali M. Gender-related factors and autoimmune pathologies.
immunes. Annales de l'institut Pasteur / Actualités. 1996;7(2): 143

22. Spector TD, Oilier W, Perry LA, Silman AJ, Thompson PW, Edwards A. Free and serum testosterone levels in 276 males: A comparative study of rheumatoid arthritis, ankylosing spondylitis and healthy controls. ClinicalRheumatology. 1989;8(1):37 41.

23. Seema C , Yashwant K, Mahendra K , Aman S ,Ranjeet B , Ranjana WM.Prevalence of autoantibodies to cellular cytoplasmic and mitotic antigens in routine antinuclear antibody reporting: Implementation of international consensus on antinuclear antibodies patterns guidelines. 2021

24. Brom M, Carrizo CE, Arana RM, Pisoni CN. Clinical description of patients with cytoplasmic discrete dots pattern (lysosome) on indirect immunofluorescence on HEp-2 cells. Clin Rheumatol. 2018;37(12):3435 7.

25. Koh WH, Dunphy J, Whyte J, Dixey J, McHugh NJ. Characterisation of anticytoplasmic antibodies and their clinical associations. Annals of the Rheumatic Diseases. 1995;54(4):269 73.

26. Lutteri L, Dierge L, Pesser M, Watrin P, Cavalier E. A paperless autoimmunity laboratory: myth or reality? Annales de Biologie Clinique. 2016;74(4):477 89.

27. Xi Q, Wu Y, Li L, Cai B, Zhang J, Yang B, et al.-Anti Mitotic Spindle Apparatus Antoantibodies: Prevalence and Disease Association in Chinese Population. J Clin Lab Anal. 2016;30(5):702 8.

28. Pieter V, Xavier B.Prevalence and clinical significance of profiles of rare antinuclear antibodies.Rev auto immune.2013;12(10)998-1003.

Summary

Introduction: Although NAA testing is frequently requested in practice, the reporting of results lacks standardization between laboratories. In the 1st international consensus on standardizing NAA nomenclature (ICAP 2014), it is recommended that cytoplasmic and mitotic spindle fluorescence be combined with nuclear fluorescence when reporting NAA results.

The aim of our study was to describe the different fluorescence aspects observed during the search for NAAs in the 1st stage and to study the clinical significance associated with the cytoplasmic marking aspects in the 2nd stage.

Material and methods: We studied all requests for NAA testing received by our laboratory during an 11-month period (January 2021- November 2021). NAA testing was performed by indirect immunofluorescence (IFI) on Hep-2 cells (EUROIMMUN® Germany).

Results: Among 2952 requests for NAA testing received during the study period, nuclear fluorescence was observed in 86% of cases, mainly speckled fluorescence (89.5%), cytoplasmic fluorescence in 8.6% of cases (14% isolated and 86% associated with nuclear fluorescence) and mitotic spindle fluorescence in 0.2% of cases. The most frequently observed aspects of cytoplasmic marking were granular (85%), reticulated (7.5%), fibrillar (4.5%), rods and rings (1.5%) and polar/golgi-like (1.5%). These aspects were associated with various clinical situations: connectivitis in 20 patients (17 cases of systemic lupus erythematosus, 2 cases of Gougerot Sjogren's syndrome and 1 case of scleroderma), diffuse interstitial lung disease in 6 patients, rheumatoid arthritis (RA) in 4 patients, polymyositis in 4 patients, dermatopolymyositis in one patient, and 1 case of primary biliary cirrhosis (PBC). Other less specific clinical situations were also observed, including mucocutaneous, articular, ocular, thromboembolic and neurological manifestations. Interestingly, three patients had a particular isolated cytoplasmic fluorescence, which prompted us to complement with specific explorations. This helped to establish the diagnoses of necrotizing myositis with anti SRP Ac in one case, anti-synthetase syndrome with anti Jo1 Ac in another, and PBC with M2-type anti-mitochondrial Ac associated with RA in the third patient.

Conclusion: Our results show a higher prevalence of nuclear and cytoplasmic fluorescence than described in the literature. The prevalence of mitotic fluorescence, on the other hand, appears to be rare. In practice, the significance of cytoplasmic fluorescence when testing for NAA is not unequivocal. Certain cytoplasmic aspects could be of real clinical interest. Hence the importance of knowing about these aspects, and mentioning them even when NAAs are negative, in order to implement techniques for identifying these Ac, when necessary, as part of a good clinical-biological collaboration.

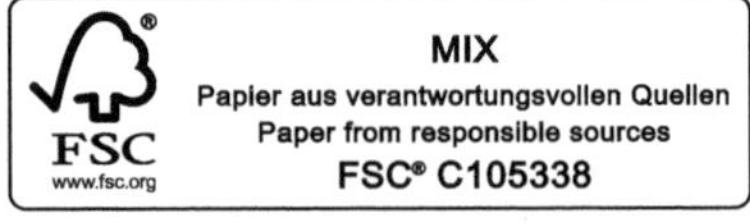

Printed by Books on Demand GmbH, Norderstedt / Germany